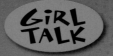
GIRL TALK

How to survive

BEING DUMPED

Lisa Miles and Xanna Eve Chown

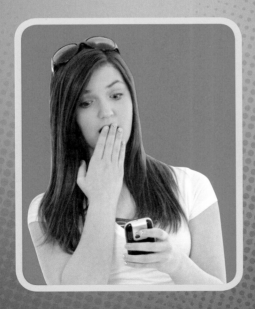

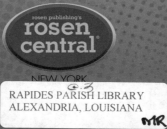
rosen publishing's
rosen central®

NEW YORK

This edition published in 2014 by:

The Rosen Publishing Group, Inc.
29 East 21st Street, New York, NY 10010

Designer: Jeni Child
Editor: Joe Harris
Consultants: Gill Lynas and Emma Hughes
Picture research: Lisa Miles and Xanna Eve Chown
With thanks to Erin Darcel
Picture credits:
All images: Shutterstock

Library of Congress Cataloging-in-Publication Data

Miles, Lisa
How to survive being dumped/[Lisa Miles and Xanna Eve Chown].—1st ed.—New York: Rosen, c2014
        p. cm.—(Girl talk)
Includes index.
ISBN: 978-1-4777-0704-3 (Library Binding)
ISBN: 978-1-4777-0716-6 (Paperback)
ISBN: 978-1-4777-0717-3 (6-pack)
1. Interpersonal relations in adolescence—Juvenile literature. 2. Teenagers—Conduct of life—Juvenile literature. 3. Rejection (psychology) in adolescence. 4. Separation (psychology)—Juvenile literature. I. Chown, Xanna Eve. II. Title.
BF724.3.I58 .M55 2014
158.'2'0835

Manufactured in China

CPSIA Compliance Information: Batch #S13YA: For further information, contact Rosen Publishing, New York, New York, at 1-800-237-9932.

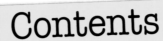

Contents

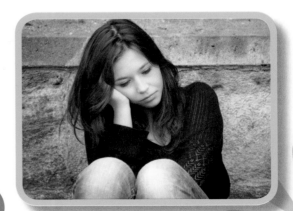

WE NEED TO talk

Your heart is in your stomach. You feel like you'll always be alone. You just can't stop crying. You've been dumped.

When someone you're really into tells you it's over, it's one of the worst feelings in the world. It's a feeling no one wants, but it will happen to most of us at some point in our lives. (Yes, it will even happen to the guy who just dumped you!)

How are you going to deal with it? Some people cry for a day and then feel better. Others take much longer. It's likely that you feel hurt, rejected, and unloved. You might keep wondering what, if anything, you did wrong – or if you will ever fall in love again.

Girl Talk is here to give you practical advice, to help you understand your emotions and to finally help you get yourself back onto your feet again.

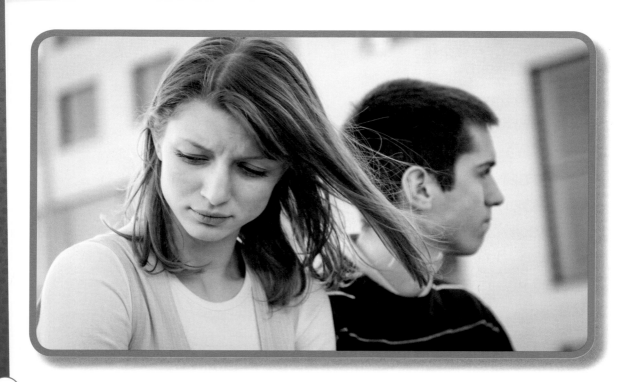

GIRL TO GIRL

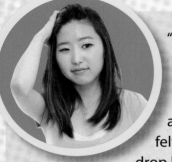

"When he said he didn't want to go out any more, I felt the floor drop beneath my feet and my heart was in my throat. How do I get over this guy fast? I don't like this feeling."

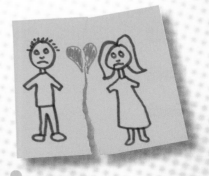

"I went out with this boy for a year and I'm still not over him. But I pretend I've moved on. I've been single for a year and a half because of it. We get along great as friends, and I've even tried to help him when he has a problem with his new girlfriend. But seeing how upset he gets over her when he wasn't at all upset over me just kills me."

"My boyfriend dumped me last night. He said he liked another girl and that she likes him, too. I am so upset about it and I can't just brush it off like my mom keeps saying. I'm really close to going to his house and begging him to take me back. I'm having a really hard time dealing with the fact that we are over."

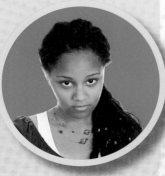

Diary

It's over!

Stories from my life

My life is officially over.

When I woke up this morning, I was happy. (Well, as happy as you can be at 7:30 on a Monday.) But now? My eyes are puffy and red and I have a headache from crying.

Jake broke up with me at lunchtime. It was super awkward. He said we needed to talk somewhere privately, so we sat on a bench as far away from everyone else as we could. But I could see everyone looking at us. He mumbled something about things not working out and taking a break for a while and that was it. I don't have a boyfriend anymore.

I don't know what to do.

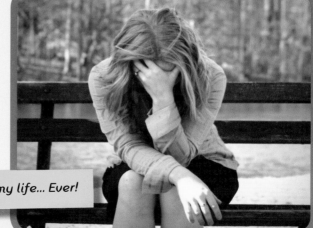

The worst day of my life... Ever!

TOP FIVE... worst ways to get dumped!

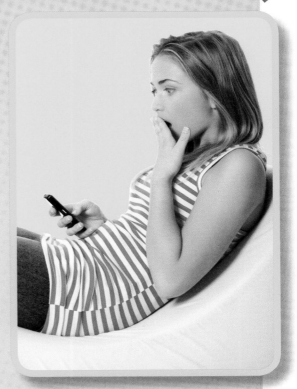

1. He sends a text that says "Sorry, babe, it's over. LOL."

2. He asks his best friend to dump you so he doesn't have to.

3. He secretly changes his Facebook relationship status to "single."

4. He gets his new girlfriend to tell you. Awkward!

5. You see pictures of him kissing a mystery girl on Facebook.

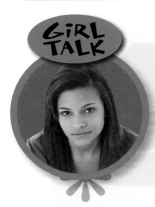

GIRL TALK

Real-life advice

Being dumped unexpectedly is a horrible shock, but with lots of time – and ice cream – things will get better! You might not believe it now, but one day you will look back on this and laugh about it.

7

FEELING down

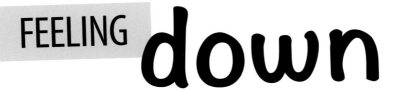

Did you know it was coming or was it a total shock to your system? Whatever happened, the fact is he's not with you any more and you are now officially single. You probably miss him and it's bound to feel strange.

Why do you feel so bad?

Your emotions will be running high right now. Which of these describes you?

* **Your pride is hurt.** You feel embarrassed because you got dumped.

* **You feel rejected.** Why didn't he want you?

* **You're confused.** He said he liked you!

* **You're jealous.** Your friend just told you he's with another girl.

* **You feel silly.** You think everyone is laughing at you for getting dumped.

* **You're SO angry.** How could he do this to you?

All about you — Emotions diary

You might feel bad now, but writing about your feelings can help you feel better in the long run. It doesn't matter how you do it – either scribble in a diary or type it into your computer – but putting things down in words can help ease the pain, give you the space to think things through, and even make you feel happier.

Put aside ten minutes each day to jot down how you feel. Make a list of all your different emotions and rate them from 1 (best) through 10 (worst). In a few weeks, things may seem better!

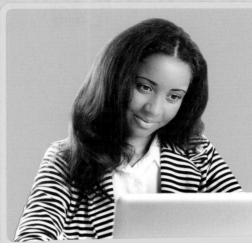

Don't worry if you don't know where to begin... just start typing and let it all out!

MONDAY

TODAY'S EMOTIONS

Embarrassed	5
Sad	8
Angry	8
Jealous	10!
Confused	4

TALKING Point

Emotions are strong feelings that affect the way you think and behave. Many people say that love is the strongest emotion. What do YOU think?

WHAT WENT wrong?

There are lots of reasons why break-ups happen. Understanding what went wrong can help you get over the pain of the split – otherwise your thoughts and emotions can spin around in circles and make you even more confused.

Different stories...

Every break-up is different and boys have viewpoints that aren't always the same as yours. If you're unsure about what happened, you could ask him for a simple reason. But don't expect a big explanation – that might not happen.

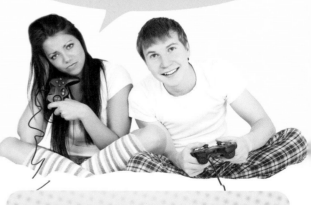

I don't like his computer games and I don't like his friends. He said I was boring!

Maybe it's a sign that you just don't have enough in common. (And don't worry, you're not boring!)

His family didn't approve of me and he felt under pressure.

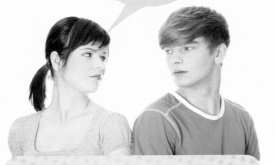

Parents and kids have strong ties, even when the kids are grown up. Sometimes people put their family's opinions first.

He decided he liked another girl more than me.

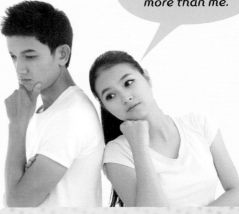

Losing out to another girl can be the hardest thing to accept. But people's feelings can change – and yours will, too!

I didn't want to go too far with him – but he didn't understand that.

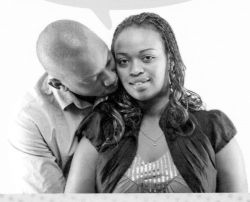

You were right to say no. If you don't feel at ease with what he wants you to do, then he's not right for you.

He said I was too clingy and he needed space.

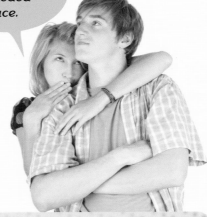

You're on a different emotional level – he wasn't ready to get serious.

WHO NEEDS friends?

When you've been dumped, the first people you turn to are your friends. They're the ones who are always going to be on your side, right? Well, that's mostly true, but friends sometimes behave in unexpected ways.

A little understanding

The chances are that your friends will be sympathetic and ready to listen – even if you cry on their shoulders for hours. If you're deciding who to talk to, you might find it easier to pick someone who's been through the same experience, as they will know where you're coming from.

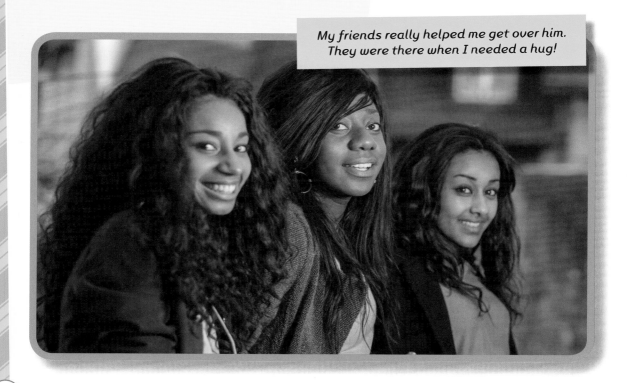

My friends really helped me get over him. They were there when I needed a hug!

Sometimes friends aren't so understanding. You might get a cold reaction or they might even gossip about you. Maybe they didn't like your boyfriend and are secretly glad you've split up. Maybe they are friends with him and have divided loyalties. Whatever the reason, if you feel like a particular friend isn't helping you, or is even being mean, then find someone else to confide in.

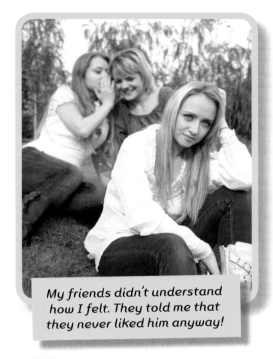

My friends didn't understand how I felt. They told me that they never liked him anyway!

Keeping it real:
Who to talk to

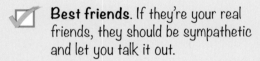
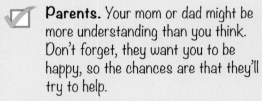

☑ **Best friends.** If they're your real friends, they should be sympathetic and let you talk it out.

☑ **Parents.** Your mom or dad might be more understanding than you think. Don't forget, they want you to be happy, so the chances are that they'll try to help.

☑ **Trusted adults.** It's sometimes hard talking to your parents but if you want grown-up advice from someone you trust, you could try one of your friends' parents, an aunt, a godparent, or a teacher.

☑ **Other help.** You might find it easier talking to someone you know less well. People such as religious leaders, your school nurse, or a guidance counselor can all help – and will listen.

GIRL TALK

Real-life advice

Friends you've been there for in the past – and you completely trust – are the best people to talk to. If this isn't possible, then your parents can be the friends you need and will help you out.

LET IT ALL out!

Talking is the best way of getting rid of bad feelings. When you tell someone how you feel, you are no longer alone with your problems. But aside from talking, there are other ways to let go of all the bad stuff!

Let it all out. But DON'T tear your hair out!

Know yourself – and your feelings

Before you can tell someone else how you feel, you have to know yourself. Recognizing your feelings is the first step to dealing with them. Admit to yourself if you feel angry, sad, or stupid. Think back to what event actually made you feel that way. Maybe it was when he got his best friend to tell you the bad news in the school playground with everyone listening.

THE LOWDOWN

Anger – is that normal?

Anger is a natural human emotion and you often feel it if you're threatened, hurt, or treated unfairly. Anger in itself is normal. However, it becomes a problem if you or someone else gets hurt because of it or if you keep on feeling angry for a long time. So get it sorted out!

When you know what your feelings are, you can tackle them. Saying, "I feel angry," either to yourself or to someone else can actually make you feel less angry!

TOP FIVE... ways to let it all out!

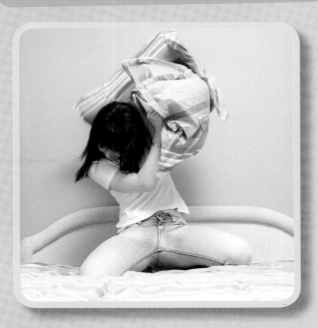

1. Punch a pillow hard, and let out your anger with a shout!

2. Scribble pages of notes and doodles about how you feel.

3. Listen to music – but pick something that doesn't remind you of HIM!

4. Breathe deeply and regularly for ten breaths and then refocus.

5. Write a quick poem – in ten lines or less! (Or maybe ten pages if you're really going for it.)

Quiz

ARE YOU ABOUT TO BE
dumped?

You've been going out for a while but you've got a sneaking suspicion that he's not happy. How do you tell if he's about to dump you? Answer the questions and see which letter you picked the most. Then check the panel opposite for your results!

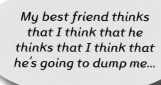

My best friend thinks that I think that he thinks that I think that he's going to dump me...

1. He's going to a party at his friend's house without you. Do you:
a) feel fine – you need to catch up on your studies anyway
b) feel nervous – he doesn't normally do that
c) feel bad – he did that last week, too (and the week before)

2. You want to see a movie but he doesn't want to. Do you:
a) find someone else to go with
b) try to persuade him, even though you know it really annoys him
c) have a huge argument about it

3. You're invited to dinner with his family. Do you:

a) feel quite excited – you like going to his place

b) feel a bit weird because you think his mom made him ask you

c) feel like refusing because you can't stand his sister

4. Before school, you see him chatting with a girl you don't know. Do you:

a) wave to him and carry on walking

b) go over and say hi – and find out who she is

c) assume he has a huge crush on her

5. He wants to go to his favorite pizza place but you hate pizza. Do you:

a) go because you know he loves it – you can always get a salad

b) go because you're scared of upsetting him

c) go and spend the whole evening sulking

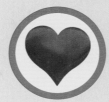

Mostly As

You two are SO into each other. Keep the balance right in your relationship and you'll stay happy!

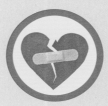

Mostly Bs

Hmm... he's acting strange. But maybe he just wants some space. Everyone needs to hang out with their own friends from time to time.

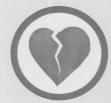

Mostly Cs

Oops – things aren't going too well, are they? Are you sure that YOU want to be in this relationship?

THE VERDICT

If you are worried about your relationship, you need to talk to him. You don't have to get into a deep conversation but he might have something on his mind or you might be imagining a problem that isn't there. And if he IS going to dump you, it's better to find out now.

Get over him!

Stories from my life

So my mom says I'll "feel better in time." But I don't know if that's true. Also, I'm not sure I want it to be true. If I get over Jake quickly, that would mean that there was never anything special between us – and I know that there was!

I haven't talked to him since we split up and that stinks. I really miss him. I'm spending a lot of time on my own, too. It's not that my friends don't want to be with me. It's just that I don't feel like hanging out with them right now. I'll only make them depressed.

I'll never be happy again!

I don't think Jake has a new girlfriend yet – so at least I know he didn't break up with me for someone else, or cheat on me behind my back. But I still don't understand why it happened. I thought we were really happy!

Will I ever get over this?

GIRL TO GIRL

"I got my heart broken and I can't stop thinking about the good times we used to have. But I've got to feel good about myself again so I can be happy – I just have to try!"

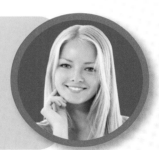

"I was the dumper – and when you're still in love with the guy it's just as hard as being dumped. I broke up with him because I was having problems at home. Breaking up with him was the hardest thing I've ever had to do."

"When I look back now, I can see that he started changing over the last few months of our relationship. When he said he saw me as just a friend it really upset me, but now I think I should have seen it coming."

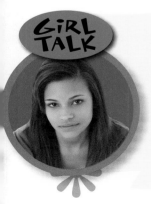

GIRL TALK

Real-life advice

You don't need to get over him quickly so don't feel you have to rush – everything takes time. Just keep an open mind and don't shut out anyone – new people always come along.

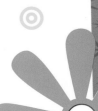

Awkward!

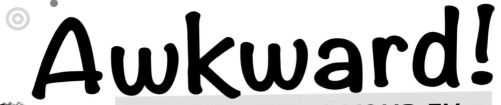

RUNNING INTO YOUR EX

Unless you were dating a guy from another part of the country, the chances are you're going to bump into each other again. Maybe it's an accidental encounter at the shopping mall or at a friend's party. Maybe you have to see him every day at school (cringe!).

OMG! We're both wearing the same sneakers! It's like we're meant to get back together!

Whatever your situation, it's a good idea to have a plan for what you're going to do when you see your ex, so that you can deal with it gracefully.

What to do – and what not to do

DON'T pretend you don't see him. That's just weird. And he'll know you're faking.

DO look amazing. If you know he's going to be at a party, you'll feel better if you look your best.

DO keep your cool. Take a deep breath, stay calm, and smile!

DON'T cry. Just don't. If you must, make sure he doesn't see you.

DON'T bring up the past by saying something like "Hi! How are you? I miss you soooo much!"

DO let him know you're fine. Mention something great that's happened recently – you saw a band, went to a cool movie, are going on holiday...

DO keep it short. There's no need for a long conversation – a quick chat is just fine.

DON'T pretend you've got a new guy to make him jealous. He might find out!

TOP FIVE... worst places to bump into your ex!

1. *Coming out of the bathroom (especially if you've been in there crying over him!)*

2. *Out shopping for underwear... with your mom.*

3. *When you stepped out to walk the dog without even brushing your hair.*

4. *In the "Feminine Hygiene" aisle at the supermarket.*

5. *When you're on a date with his best friend... (Oops!)*

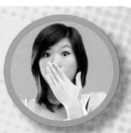

HOW TO GET
over him

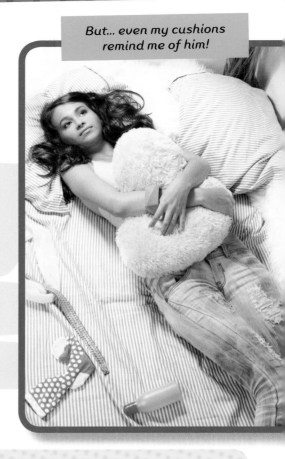

But... even my cushions remind me of him!

I t takes time to get over a break-up. Sadly, you can't just go to bed and sleep for weeks until you feel better – however much you may want to! So, while you're still getting over him, here are some tried-and-true ways to get back on track.

MAKE A LIST

Write down all the things that you didn't like about him. Every time you read them think how lucky you are to be away from someone with such annoying habits!

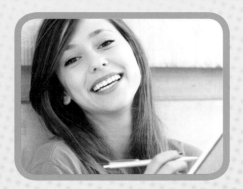

TIME TO CRY

All you want to do is stay in bed, eat chocolate, watch sad movies, and cry. Fine – it's good to let it out. Make sure you give yourself enough time to grieve – but then move on!

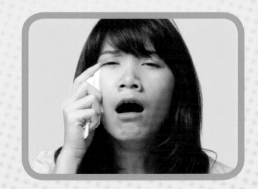

STAY BUSY

Stop moping around the house and organize things to keep you occupied instead. Spend as much time with friends and family as you can. The more fun you are having, the less likely you are to be thinking about him all the time!

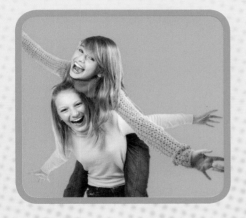

DON'T PHONE

Calling him or replaying his phone messages just so that you can hear his voice will not help you heal. Plus, you'll be super-sensitive to whatever he is saying. This means that he might hurt you again without meaning to.

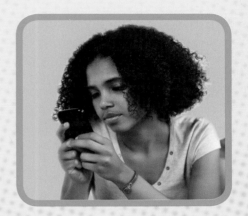

KEEP TALKING

Don't feel guilty about opening up to your friends. You'd be there for them, too, right? It always helps to share the way you feel with people who are on your side.

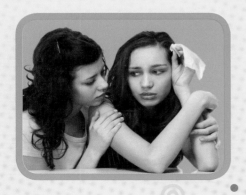

THE LOWDOWN

Crying is good for you

Why? Tears remove toxins that have built up in your body thanks to stress. Plus, crying is proven to help lift your mood and lower your stress levels!

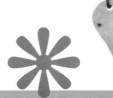

23

Get rid
OF HIM

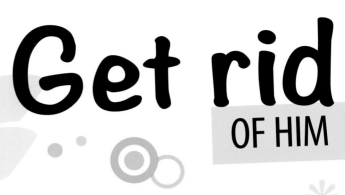

He's not around any more but his T-shirt is... and his baseball cap... and the old Valentine's card he sent you. Be brave – getting rid of his stuff will help you to get rid of him!

It's just stuff

It's great to keep mementos of the past – but only if they make you happy when you look at them. So if his old T-shirt makes you cry, give it back to him – along with anything else you borrowed such as books, music, or gadgets.

The hardest things to get rid of are the cute, romantic things. Throw away the Valentine's card and delete his emails and messages from your phone – even the adorable ones! You might have to be a little bit hard on yourself, but reminding yourself about him all the time won't help you to get over him.

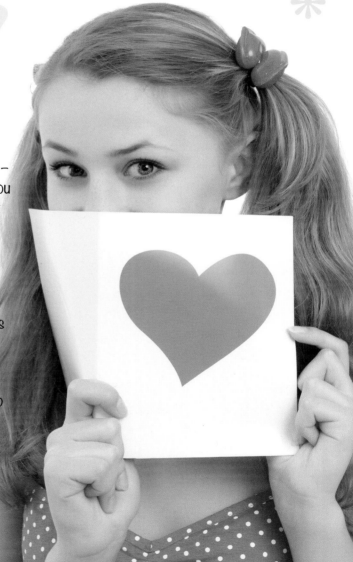

All about you | Make a memory box

If there's anything that you really can't bear to part with, such as the birthday card he made for you or a really cute photo, then you could pack it away with your other mementos or stick it in a scrapbook.

Put everything you want to keep in a box and put it away somewhere that's hard to get at, such as at the back of a cupboard or in an attic. You can look at that birthday card some other time when you feel better, but don't have it sitting on your desk!

Throw it away or put it away – just don't keep looking at it!

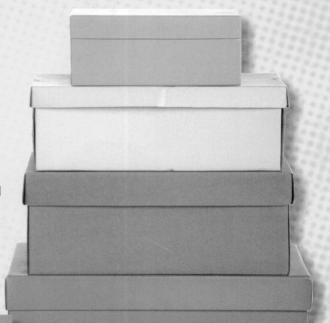

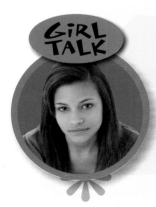

GIRL TALK

Real-life advice

Deleting texts and getting rid of any little gifts he gave you is a vital step in moving on. Remember, you can't live in the present if you're dreaming about the past.

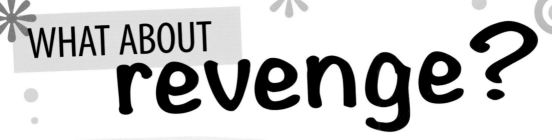

WHAT ABOUT revenge?

Do you fantasize about finding a way to totally embarrass him in front of his friends?

Stop!

Revenge isn't a good idea. When the heat of the moment has died down, you are not going to feel good about yourself. The best way to get revenge on your ex is to be happy without him. Let him see that you are living the best life ever – and he is not even a tiny part of it.

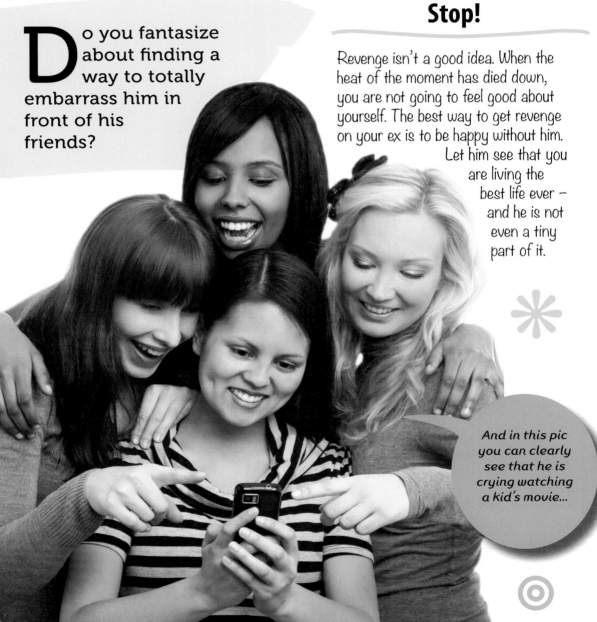

And in this pic you can clearly see that he is crying watching a kid's movie...

TOP FIVE... worst break-ups in history!

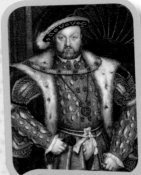

1. *Actress Elizabeth Taylor was mega-famous for breaking up with people. She got married eight times – twice to the same man!*

2. *Britney Spears married childhood friend Jason Allen Alexander. The marriage was over 55 hours later.*

3. *Edward VIII couldn't marry his true love, Wallis Simpson, and be King of England. So he broke up… with the monarchy, rather than Wallis!*

4. *In the 16th century, King Henry VIII had six wives whose fate was recorded in a rhyme: divorced, beheaded, died, divorced, beheaded, survived.*

5. *Medea – a woman from Greek mythology – sent her ex's new wife a dress that burned her alive, then escaped on a chariot pulled by…er… dragons.**

* Don't try this at home.

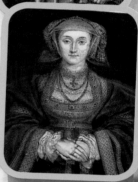

King Henry VIII and his fourth wife, Anne of Cleves.

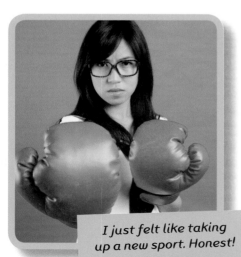

I just felt like taking up a new sport. Honest!

TALKING *Point*

Do you know anyone who has taken revenge on an ex? Did it work out well for them? Who did you feel more sorry for?

ARE YOU over him?

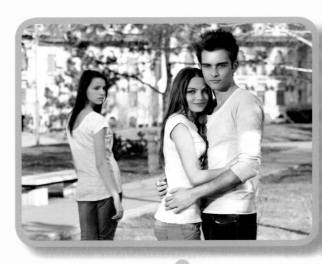

So... are you over him yet? Take this quiz and follow the arrows to find out.

Would you invite him to your best friend's party?
YES
NO

START HERE!

Do you still think about him a lot?
NO
YES

Do you have pictures of him on your wall?
NO
YES

Do you get nervous when you talk to him?
YES
NO

Do you try to be in places you might bump into each other?
NO
YES

Do you think you'll get back together?
NO
YES

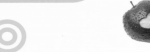

WOW!

You are officially over him. Doesn't it feel great? You go, girl!

Do you feel ready to date again?

YES

NO

HMMM!

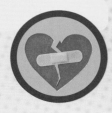

You're nearly over him but you need a bit more time before you totally move on.

Do your friends think you talk about him too much?

NO

YES

UH-OH!

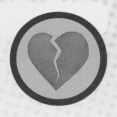

You are so not over him yet. Go back and look at some of the earlier pages!

Do you ever dream about him?

YES

NO

Would you change **anything** to get him back?

NO

YES

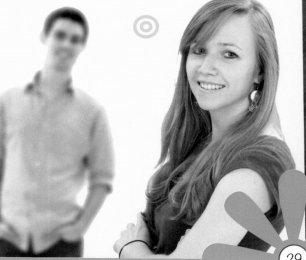

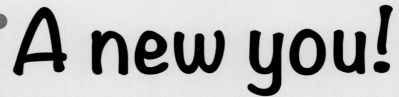

A new you!

Stories from my life

Last night I went out with Sophie and you know what? I didn't think about Jake all evening – not even once! Total result.

It was stupid of me not to talk to my friends about how I was feeling. As soon as I let them know they were all really sympathetic and wanted to help. We all went out for a burger and everyone shared stories about their ex-boyfriends.

Anyway, I feel a lot better now. I can even walk past Jake in the corridor at school and say "hi." I don't stop to talk – that would be too embarrassing right now – but maybe someday we can be friends again.

Sophie told me she thinks her friend Ryan would be just right for me and wants to introduce us. He sounds cool, but I'm not sure I want another relationship right now. I'm having too much fun hanging out with my friends again!

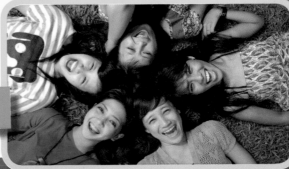

Time to get happy!

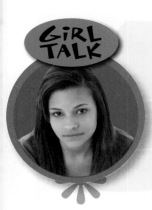

GIRL TALK

Real-life advice

Never underestifriend the power of good friends! There's no rush to find a new guy – so take things as slowly as you like. Remember, whatever happens with boys, you still have your trusted girlfriends!

GIRL TO GIRL

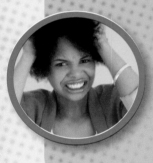

"Remember the good times you had together and look at the whole thing as a good experience. You'll feel bad at first, but try to come to terms with the fact that he's gone."

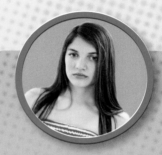

"I heard that the time you take to get over someone depends on the amount of time you were together. I don't know. I think everyone's different though and you can't plan things like that! Some people get over things quickly, others take time."

"Spend time with your friends and enjoy being by yourself, too! When you're busy laughing with your friends or wrapped up in a book, you won't even notice you're missing him!"

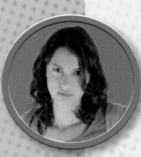

HAPPY TO be you!

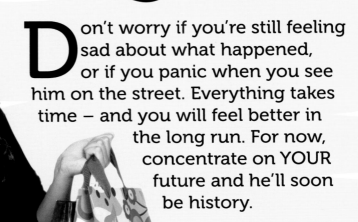

Don't worry if you're still feeling sad about what happened, or if you panic when you see him on the street. Everything takes time – and you will feel better in the long run. For now, concentrate on YOUR future and he'll soon be history.

Being single rocks!

If you've been neglecting your friends, now is the time to reconnect with them. They'll understand why they haven't seen you around for a while so don't be shy – invite them over for a girly night in or let them know about that movie you've been desperate to see (that HE didn't want to!).

You can now spend your weekends shopping with your sister or chatting with your best friend, instead of watching him at football practice. You have the freedom to be yourself – so enjoy it!

> I spent so much time with HIM that I almost forgot how much I love hanging out with my sister.

TOP FIVE...
ways you know you are over him

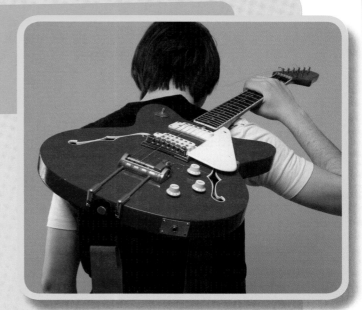

1. *It's bedtime – and you haven't thought about him all day.*

2. *You walked past his favorite pizza place without looking in the window.*

3. *You heard "your" song on the radio and didn't cry.*

4. *You mentioned his name without feeling weird.*

5. *The guy with the guitar on the bus this morning looked kind of cute.*

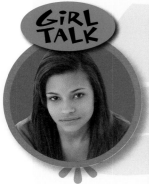

GiRL TALK

Real-life advice

When you're single you can catch up with all the little things you did with your girlfriends that you might have missed – like dancing around to silly songs and making up code names for the cutest boys in your class.

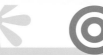

33

IT'S TIME TO move on

Now you're single, how do you know when it's the right time to start dating someone else? The last thing you want is to go out with a guy when you're really not ready for it. That spells trouble!

Mixed feelings

You know your old relationship is over, but you might have mixed feelings about dating again. Part of you might want to have a new boyfriend but part of you might feel scared in case you get hurt. And how do you know if the new guy is the right person?

Those feelings are all completely normal. One way to sort things out is to dip a toe in the water. Go out on a date, keep it casual for a while, and see how things develop.

On the other hand, if nobody special has come along and you are happy being single, then why not stay that way for a while? Having a boyfriend isn't necessary and if you're happy on your own that's OK, too.

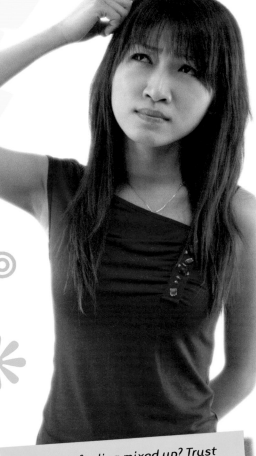

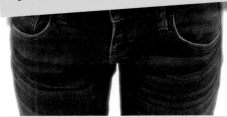

Are you feeling mixed up? Trust your instincts – you'll know when you're ready to start dating again.

Keeping it real:

Knowing you're ready to date

☑ **You've got things together.** You've got friends, stuff to keep you busy, and you're enjoying what you do. You have a life outside of being someone's girlfriend! Having said that, a date might be fun.

☑ **Crush!** Having a crush on a new guy is a telltale sign you're ready to date. You're having feelings for someone else, so why not follow your heart and have a little fun?

☑ **Boys notice you.** Are you getting a lot of male attention? Maybe without even knowing it, you're giving off signals that you're interested in dating. If a boy asks you out and you think he's attractive, why not give it a try?

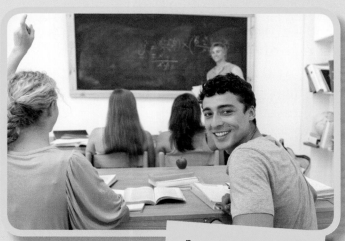

Does he keep asking you to be his partner in class? He's noticed you!

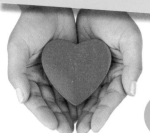

THE LOWDOWN

On the rebound?

When someone is "on the rebound" it means that she's still hung up on her ex. She might go out with other people in an effort to get over the ex, but it often doesn't work out. So if you still have feelings for Mr. Wrong, it's best not to start searching for Mr. Right just yet!

ARE YOU dumping him?

When someone dumps you, you're suddenly single – you don't have a choice in the matter. But what if you're the one who wants to end the relationship? It's not always easy making that BIG decision...

Air guitar fail! He's got to go.

Be honest

It can be hard to be completely honest with yourself, let alone with someone else, but if you're dating a guy and any of these things apply then it's time to move on:

* **You don't want to be on your own** – so you're staying with him.

* **You're bored by his conversation** – do you really have to hear about his favorite band again?

* **You're always arguing** – over every little thing.

* **He's not making you happy** – and you're not making him happy either.

* **It's getting too heavy** – he follows you around everywhere and you need some space.

* **You feel sorry for him** – and that's the only reason you're with him.

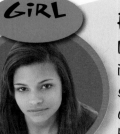

GiRL

Real-life advice

It's not a good idea to stay with someone you don't want to be with because you're too scared to dump them! Better for both of you to be brave and end it.

Keeping it real:
Break-up basics

You've made the decision – so how do you tell him the news?

☒ **DON'T** text him or message him on Facebook. That's the easy way out.

☒ **DON'T** get your best friend to tell him. That's embarrassing for both of them.

☒ **DON'T** tell him in front of his friends. That makes you look bad.

☒ **DON'T** tell him on his birthday. That's just mean.

☑ **DO** tell him yourself and face-to-face if you can – that way you can talk it through quickly and it's better for both of you.

☑ **DO** tell him when you're alone – and not at school. Pick a time and a place where he can go and think it over in his own time.

☑ **DO** be honest but polite. Ripping someone's personality to shreds is never nice.

☑ **DO** keep calm. If he gets upset just keep it short – and get out of the situation as fast as you can!

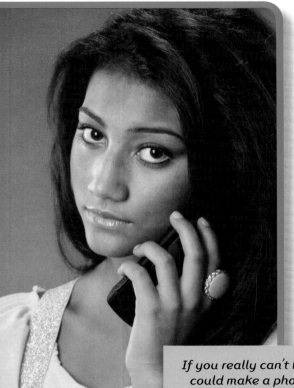

If you really can't bear to see him face-to-face, you could make a phone call with the bad news – and that way you can still follow the break-up basics.

ARE YOU ON THE
rebound?

Have you been super-quick to get involved with someone new after your break-up? Even though you might not be totally into them? It's better than being on your own, right? Hmm.

This sounds like a rebound relationship! Some rebound relationships work out but most don't, and they can be even more destructive than the earlier break-up. Try this quiz to see if you're on the rebound. Give yourself one point every time you say "yes" to one of the questions on the next page.

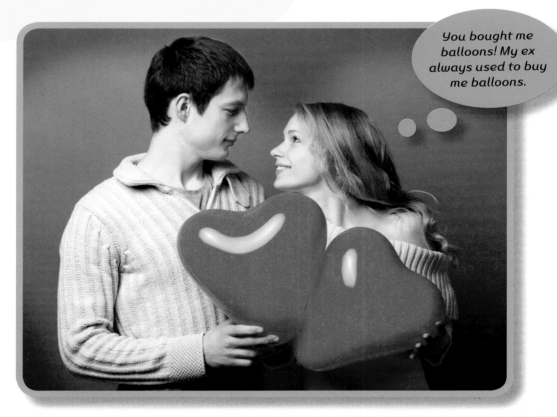

You bought me balloons! My ex always used to buy me balloons.

1. Did you break up with your ex less than a month ago?

2. Do you think that deep down your ex wants you back?

3. Do you compare other guys with your ex?

4. Have you been out with only one other guy since your split?

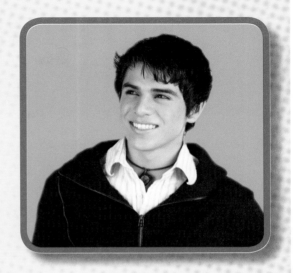

5. Do you have crushes on lots of different guys at once?

6. Do you feel jealous if you hear your ex is spending time with another girl?

7. If you picture yourself out on a date, is it with your ex?

8. If you have a good time with a new guy do you feel guilty?

9. Do you date people who are just like your ex?

10. If you were on a date and your ex phoned, would you take the call?

1 – 3 points

You are over your ex and ready to start dating if you want to. In fact, it wouldn't be surprising if you were out on a date right now! Um… you might want to hide this book.

4 – 7 points

You're enjoying being single but you're not ready to start dating yet. That's fine – take your time and wait for Mr. Right to come along. There's no need to hurry!

8 – 10 points

You think you're over him but you're not! You're on the rebound, so any guy you are dating is always going to be second best to your memories. Eek! Take a bit more time.

Boy talk
FROM HIS POINT OF VIEW

Breaking up is tough on boys, too. In some ways, it can be worse than it is for girls. It is far more socially acceptable for girls to talk about their emotions, whereas boys are more likely to hear, "Get over it. She wasn't worth it," or, "There's plenty more fish in the sea," from their friends.

Mixed messages

How a guy acts after the break-up can be confusing. He might say he wants to be friends but then ignore you on the street. Here's what might be going on in his head:

✳ **Acting mean** – if he is being really obnoxious after a break-up, it usually means the split was hard on him and he is lashing out.

✳ **Going cold** – he's acting like he doesn't know you and it makes you feel terrible. Either he's trying not to get hurt or he's worried that the split is hard on you, too.

✳ **New girl** – he didn't wait more than two seconds before finding a new relationship. It sounds like he's looking for a way out of having to deal with what happened.

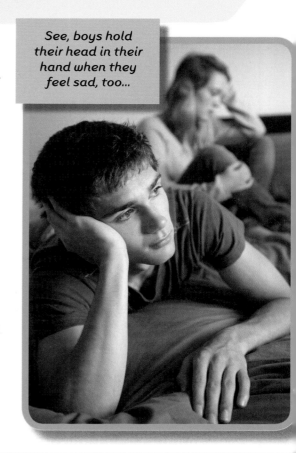

See, boys hold their head in their hand when they feel sad, too...

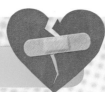

BOYS SAY...

"I'm a nice guy. But girls are always dumping me for some jerk who just leaves them in a week. Girls are always asking where the nice guys are – I can tell them! But nice guys might turn into jerks when they get dumped for a jerk."

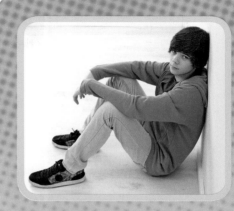

"My ex dumped me on my Facebook wall. Can you believe that? We had been friends for three years before we got together. I stuck to my hobbies and friends and eventually I forgot about her. But it took a really long time."

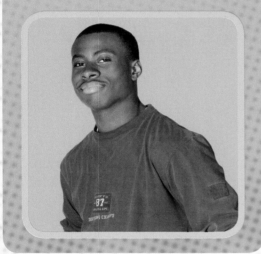

"My girlfriend told me she loved me on the phone. Then, the next day she got her friend to dump me for her. I was devastated and my heart was totally broken. I still don't know why she dumped me. Maybe I will never know and that hurts."

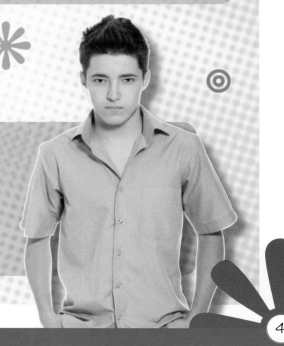

HEALTHY you!

There's a lot more to being healthy than just your physical well-being. Your mental health, emotional state, and your physical wellness all affect your general health.

Feeling stressed?

Everyone copes with problems differently, even if they are going through a similar experience. This is due to personality, circumstances, and support from family and friends.

If you've just broken up with someone, you're bound to feel a mixture of emotions. Whatever your situation, an emotional upheaval can lead to stress – and that's not good! Common signs of stress include:

* headaches and tension
* constant worrying
* irritability and losing your temper
* feeling stuck in a rut
* feeling unsociable
* difficulty concentrating at school
* eating too much or too little

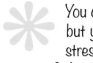

You can't change what has happened, but you can change the way that you deal with stressful situations, which in turn can bring back feelings of happiness. Top stress-beating tips include:

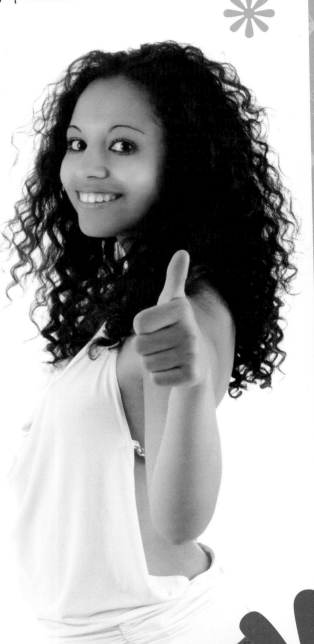

* **Learning how to relax** – have a warm bath, read, do some exercise, listen to music, do something that makes you happy!

* **Talking to someone** – share your problems with a friend, parent, or other adult who is responsible for you.

* **Eating and drinking well** – make sure you don't skip meals or overeat, and drink plenty of water.

* **Sleeping well** – tiredness makes you less able to beat stress, so get a full-night's sleep every night.

* **Avoiding stressful situations whenever you can** – for example, if you know that he goes to the mall every Friday night, avoid going there yourself for a while until you can cope better.

THE LOWDOWN

Watch what you drink!

Drinks that contain caffeine – such as tea, coffee, cola, and energy drinks – stop you from relaxing. This can overtax your body and add to your stress levels. Check the packaging to see how much caffeine your drink contains!

FAQs

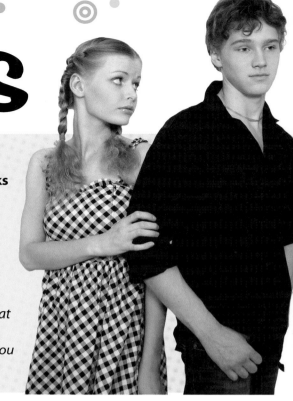

Q I was totally gutted when my boyfriend dumped me four weeks ago. I thought I was over him… then he asked me out again! Should I go back?

A *Your ex sounds confused. Does he genuinely think he made a mistake or is he just messing with you? If you can both sit down and figure out what went wrong before, you may be able to work things out. But be careful – you may end up getting hurt again.*

Q My boyfriend just dumped me and asked my best friend out instead. She told me she wants to date him but won't if it upsets me. It does! But I feel bad saying no.

A *Your best friend has put you in a tricky position. Dating your friend's ex is not very cool and she knows it – that's why she asked for your permission! If your ex and your best friend are really into each other it's going to be hard to stop them from getting together. They might end up sneaking around behind your back – which would make you feel terrible. Why not ask your friend if she can give you a bit of time to get over him before she starts anything?*

Q I think my boyfriend wants to dump me. He's not said anything, but we're spending less time together and things just feel different. I don't want to ask him in case he does dump me. What can I do?

A *The only way to deal with this is to talk to him and ask him what is going on. It's not easy, but you will have to be brave. If he does tell you that it's over it will hurt – but it can't be worse than spending all your time worrying about what he might be thinking.*

Q My boyfriend started spreading really bad rumors around the school about me after he dumped me. They're totally made up – help!

A *Spreading rumors is a form of bullying. You need to talk to him and fast. Tell him that what he is doing is wrong and hurtful. Ask him to clear your name. You can also tell a teacher or guidance counselor. They will take a very serious approach to what is going on.*

Q The best friend of my ex asked me out. I think he's all right, but I only really want to date him to make my ex feel bad. Is that OK?

A *I think you know that it's not OK. You are misleading your ex's friend into thinking that you really like him when you don't AND you are deliberately trying to hurt your ex. However bad your ex was when he dumped you, you don't have to stoop to this level. Plus this is the sort of plan that always ends up backfiring – on you. It's safer to stay away.*

Q It's been weeks since we split up, but I really can't get over my ex. I can't eat or sleep and sometimes feel like hurting myself.

A *This is serious and you need to talk to someone you trust, such as a parent or a teacher. Your doctor can also offer support in managing these feelings. Remember – you don't have to go through this alone.*

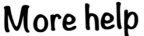

More help

If you have a question that has not been addressed here, you might want to check out the further reading and Web sites sections on page 47.

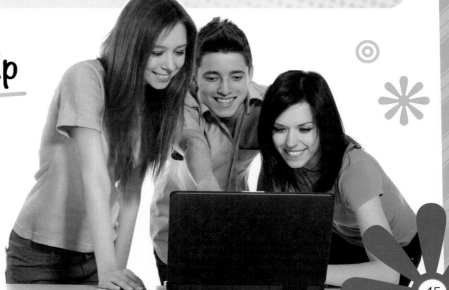

45

Glossary

counselor A person qualified to give you advice and help in situations where you find it hard to cope.

dumped No longer being in a relationship, because your girlfriend or boyfriend has decided to end it.

embarrassment Feeling a sense of shame about something that you have done, or something that has happened to you.

grieving Feeling sad about the loss of someone or something.

loyalty Feeling faithful toward someone or something and being prepared to stand up for him or her, no matter what.

mental health The well-being of your mind. This is just as important as the health of your body!

mislead To deliberately give someone an untrue impression about something.

monarchy A form of government where a king or queen rules over a country.

mope To behave in a constantly gloomy way, without any energy or enthusiasm.

mythology Stories featuring gods and monsters that belong to a culture or religious tradition.

obnoxious Highly offensive or annoying.

pressuring Forcing a person to do something when they don't really want to.

rebound To move quickly from one relationship to another.

reconnect To make contact with someone you have not spoken to in a while.

reject To refuse to accept someone or something that is being offered to you.

revenge Causing hurt or harm to someone in return for something that they have done to you.

stress A physical response to events that make you feel threatened or upset your balance. A little stress is good as it helps us meet challenges. A lot of stress can damage your quality of life and your health.

toxins Poisons produced within living cells in your body. Your body can break them down and get them out of your body in different ways, for example through your pores when you sweat.

unsociable Not wanting to spend time with friends or engaged in friendly social relations.

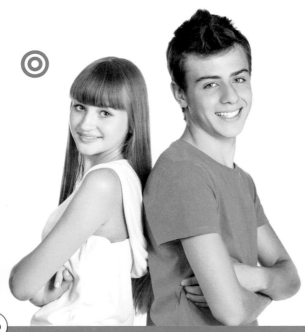

Get help!

There are places to go to if you need more help. The following books and Web sites will give you more information and advice.

Further reading

The Rough Guide to Girl Stuff by Kaz Cooke (Rough Guides, 2009)

The 6 Most Important Decisions You'll Ever Make: A Guide for Teens by Sean Covey (Touchstone, 2006)

The Truth About Breaking Up, Making Up, and Moving On by Chad Eastham (Thomas Nelson, 2013)

The Truth About Guys by Chad Eastham (Thomas Nelson, 2012)

Your First Boyfriend by Katie Hentges (Rosen Publishing, 2012)

What Your Mother Never Told You: A Teenage Girls Survival Guide by Richard M. Dudum (Booksurge Publishing, 2007)

Web sites

Due to the changing nature of Internet links, Rosen Publishing has developed an online list of Web sites related to the subject of this book. This site is updated regularly. Please use this link to access the list:

http://www.rosenlinks.com/GTALK/Dump

Index

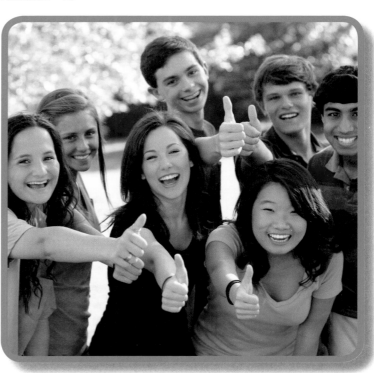

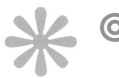